THE FERTILITY Question

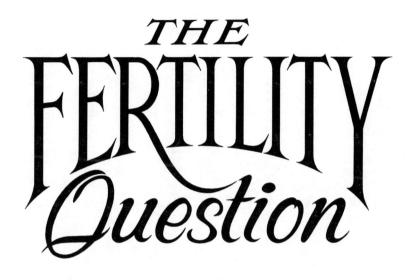

THE FERTILITY Question

Margaret Nofziger

THE BOOK PUBLISHING COMPANY

SUMMERTOWN, TENNESSEE

ISBN 0-913990-43-4

Printed in the USA.

FOREWORD

Infertile couples make up the largest silent minority in the world today, as one in six couples has difficulty conceiving. This well-written book gives excellent information on the problems an infertile woman may encounter, with a particularly good discussion on taking and interpreting the basal temperature. Understanding one's anatomy and physiology is of particular value for the infertile couple, and Ms. Nofziger's discussions on ovulation and the menstrual cycle are both accurate and easy to understand.

I highly recommend this book for all persons interested in a brief, clear discussion of female infertility.

James F. Daniell, M.D.
Department of Obstetrics and Gynecology
Division of Reproductive Endocrinology
Vanderbilt University Medical Center
Nashville, Tennessee

TABLE OF CONTENTS

FEMALE REPRODUCTIVE ORGANS

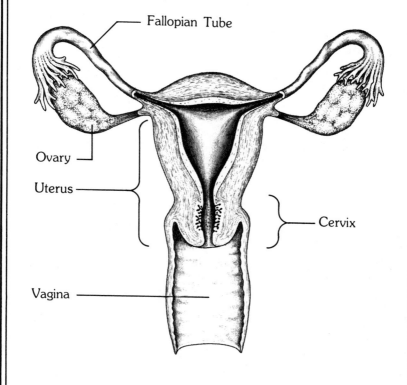

Fallopian Tube

Ovary

Uterus

Cervix

Vagina

THE FERTILITY QUEST

Here you are, investigating your fertility. Your doctor or your own curiosity has led you toward a detailed study of your reproductive potential.

Your goal is CONCEPTION, a process taken for granted by most, sought with passion by some. Conception occurs when an egg from the woman meets and merges with a sperm from the man in the outer segment of her fallopian tube. Then the combined entity continues on to implant in the uterus. Conception is not necessarily automatic. For a few people, it is instantaneous the first time they make love; but this is the exception, not the rule. If you don't conceive the first few cycles you try, it doesn't mean much. Not everyone conceives that easily. It usually takes a few months for anyone of ordinary fertility to become pregnant.

There is a "normal bell curve" of fertility. Couples are not just fertile or infertile. Some are "superfertile." Their combination of good sperm count, very supportive cervical mucus, etc., makes them conceive very readily. Other people have a combination of fertility factors leading to an "average" fertility, and others, to a reduced fertility to a greater or lesser degree.

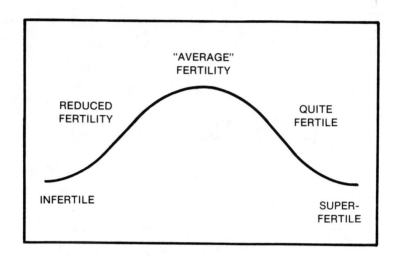

The female half of a couple's fertility depends primarily on the phenomenon of OVULATION, the eruption of an egg from the ovary. Ovulation is very basic to fertility. Early in your study, you can observe your Basal Body Temperature (BBT) in order to establish whether and when you ovulate.

The Basal Temperature Chart is the doctor's first test in an infertility workup. It involves recording your waking temperature daily for about three months. You can do this with your doctor's help, or on your own, previous to a formal workup. Sometimes family planning clinics offer infertility counseling, screening, and referral. Whatever your approach, you will need to observe your BBT. It is a valid scientific test for ovulation and problems concerning ovulation. This book will instruct you in recording and interpreting your chart.

While you are charting your temperature, you can also observe and learn about your cervical mucus, a normal female discharge that changes in quantity and character according to the hormones secreted by the ovary. The mucus will confirm and extend the information from the basal temperature.

The FERTILITY AWARENESS thus gained will also help you in understanding yourself at a deep biological/psychological level. Acknowledging and exploring your cyclic nature is an experience unto itself—a scientific journey through yourself, taking notes along the way.

If you can establish by your charts that ovulation does occur, even if infrequently, then some special attention to the timing of intercourse may be helpful, provided there are not insurmountable problems with the fallopian tubes, that there are sperm present, etc. (A low sperm count can be helped by "timing"—saving up precious sperm before the most fertile days of the female cycle.)

Of course, there are many factors that can contribute to apparent infertility; and often, it is a combination of several factors that predisposes a couple to have difficulty conceiving a child. We will discuss these factors and their diagnostic tests. And we will explore in detail the female fertility cycle with its special road map—the BBT chart—for signs of THE EGG. THE SPERM, being the other half of the germinating package, will need some investigation also. But this book is written primarily to assist you, the woman, since your reproductive capacity is both more complicated and more apt to benefit from personal study. This book is about ovulation and you.

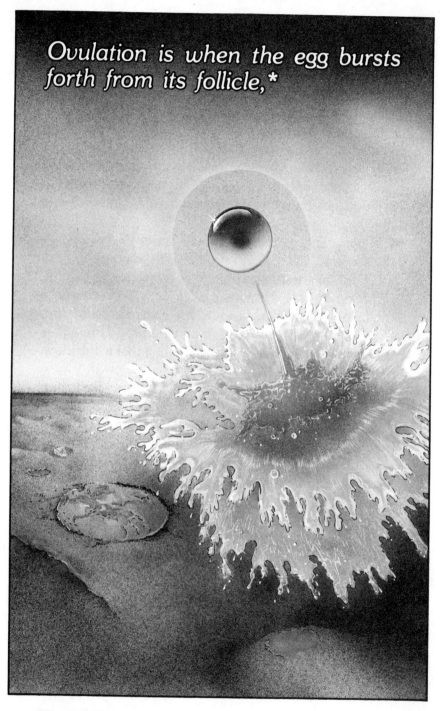

Ovulation is when the egg bursts forth from its follicle,*

*The fluid-filled sac on the ovary that held and nourished the egg as it ripened and matured.

to travel down the fallopian tube,

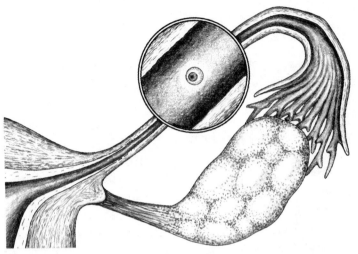

possibly meeting the sperm, and

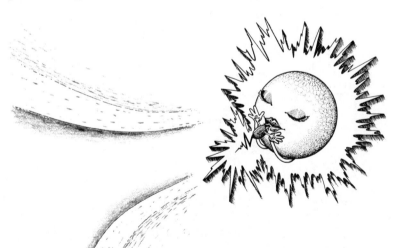

on to the uterus.

THE CYCLE

THE CYCLE

To study your reproductive capacity, you need to first become familiar with your CYCLE of ovulation and menstruation, and with the terms used to locate points in time within that cycle. The menstrual periods are the most obvious signposts of a complex dance of hormones controlling female fertility.

The female fertility cycle is a repeating course of events. It starts with the build-up of the lining of the uterus in preparation to receive an egg from the ovary; next is the coming and going of the egg; and it ends with menstruation—the shedding of the uterine lining.

The *average* length of women's cycles is 28 days, but this does not mean that most women have 28 day cycles. It means that some have 26 day cycles, some have 24 or 25, many have 29 or 30, and some have 35 days or more.

The cycle consists of all the days from one period to the next, starting with the first day of the period and ending with the day before the start of the following period.

So now you know basic reference points and can get your bearings when you hear your doctor or clinic counselor talk about the "day of the cycle," or "day 12," or "the beginning of the cycle," or "near the end of the cycle."

Ovulation is caused each cycle by:

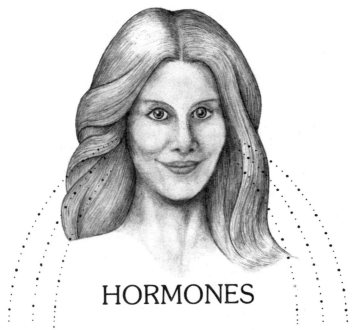

HORMONES

The endocrine hormones that determine your cycle come from the anterior (front) portion of the pituitary gland (which is in the center of your head) and from the ovaries themselves.

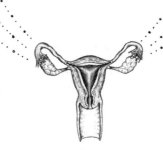

THE HORMONE SEQUENCE THAT CAUSES THE FEMALE CYCLE GOES LIKE THIS:

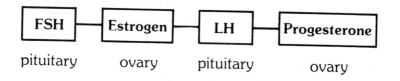

FSH	Estrogen	LH	Progesterone
pituitary	ovary	pituitary	ovary

1. The pituitary gland in the center of your head is stimulated by some special hormone substances from the hypothalamus (a part of the brain) to release the Follicle Stimulating Hormone (FSH) into the bloodstream.

2. FSH stimulates the follicles of the ovary to ripen an egg.

3. As the follicles begin to ripen, and the eggs grow, the follicles release a hormone called *estrogen* into the bloodstream.

4. Rising levels of estrogen cause the uterine lining to begin to thicken and tell the pituitary to release another hormone called Luteinizing Hormone (LH), which ultimately causes ovulation of the most mature egg.

5. After the egg is released from the ovary, a little crater is left where the egg's follicle used to be. This little crater is called the *corpus luteum*. The corpus luteum secretes the temperature-raising hormone, *progesterone*, into the bloodstream. Progesterone causes the lining of the womb to further thicken and ripen in preparation for a possible pregnancy. (The lining of the womb would feed and sustain the embryo until its placenta was functioning.)

This little temporary endocrine gland, the corpus luteum, doesn't last forever. It only has a short lifespan of about 12 to 16 days.

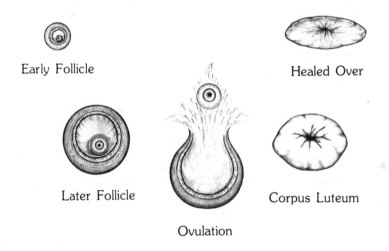

Early Follicle

Healed Over

Later Follicle

Corpus Luteum

Ovulation

At the end of its function, the corpus luteum shrivels up and becomes a scar on the ovary. The progesterone secretion stops, and hence, the period begins.

THE TIMELINE OF YOUR CYCLE

It is the time of ovulation that determines the onset of the following period as a result of the lifespan of the corpus luteum. This gland has a temporary lifespan of approximately a fortnight, or 12-16 days. When it heals over, the progesterone stops and the period commences.

The limited, regular lifespan of the corpus luteum is the reason for the fairly constant length of the "after ovulation" phase of the cycle; but the segment *before* ovulation can vary according to the length of the cycle.

Long cycles will have a late ovulation and short cycles will have an early ovulation.

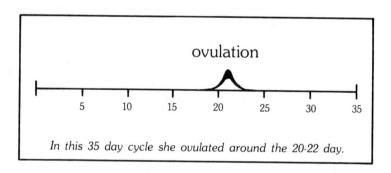

In this 35 day cycle she ovulated around the 20-22 day.

Ovulation happens about two weeks before the following period. (Not 14 days after the previous period.) It can happen anywhere from 12-16 days before, but mostly around 14 days before.

A MATTER OF TIMING

Sometimes the apparent inability to conceive is simply a matter of timing; a couple might be missing the short time each cycle in which conception is possible.

There are really only about four days each cycle when conception can occur. Obviously, you could conceive on the day of ovulation (if the fallopian tubes are open, sperm abundant, etc.). But the egg only lives for 12 to 24 hours after it pops out of the follicle. If it popped at 6:30 AM and lived until 7:30 PM, and you made love at 10:00 PM, it would be too late *for that whole cycle.*

The lifespan of the egg represents one of the four possibly fertile days. What about the other three? Well, sperm have a lifespan of 2 or 3 days (possibly 4, but not likely). If you made love on Monday and ovulated on Wednesday, the egg would be fresh and the sperm would be in there, ready and waiting. (Of course, if the tubes are blocked or the sperm too few, even these four days may not be fertile.) So, if you make love infrequently, whether by habit or because of job circumstances, or just coincidentally at the wrong time, you might miss the fertile times of each cycle for months or years. If this was the only problem, you would probably eventually conceive.

Many women can be helped to conceive by becoming more aware of their fertility cycle with its limited opportunities for conception.

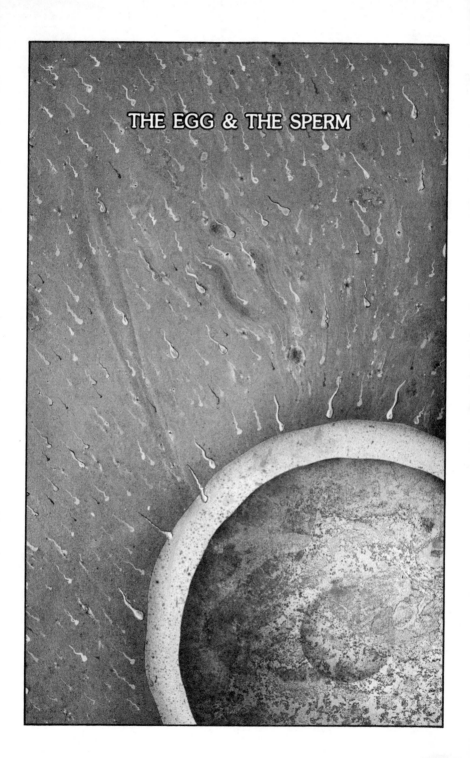

CAUSES OF REDUCED FERTILITY OR INFERTILITY

There are many causes of subfertility or infertility. The main causes are scarred fallopian tubes, low sperm count, and problems with ovulation.

SCARRED FALLOPIAN TUBES

Sometimes the fallopian tubes are blocked with scar tissue from a previous infection. Scarred fallopian tubes can cause a mechanical blockage of the tube, preventing the sperm from reaching the egg and/or the fertilized egg from reaching the womb.

Scarring can be caused by an acute infection of the uterus and tubes, or a chronic infection known as Pelvic Inflammatory Disease—PID. Infecting organisms can enter the uterus through the vagina and cause this condition. Infection can spread through the tubes, scarring them, and out into the abdominal cavity. PID is often hard to cure completely, even with modern antibiotics. Another source of infection that can cause scar tissue in the tubes and PID is, of course, gonorrhea.

Sometimes scar tissue from a uterine and tubal infection or PID can cause the end of the tube nearest to the ovary (the fimbriated end) to become attached to the ovary itself. This can cause subfertility or infertility because the fimbriated end of the tube is supposed to be able to move freely. It has a special ability and function to envelop the specific part of

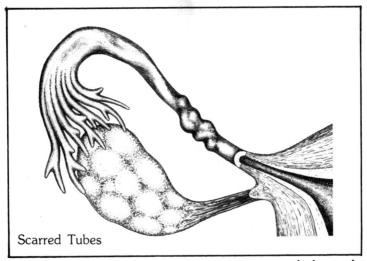

Scarred Tubes

the ovary where the egg is emerging, and through gentle motion, guide the egg into the tube.

There are three tests available to diagnose tubal occlusion. The two "office" tests are the Rubin test and hydrotubation. The Rubin test is considered obsolete by many doctors because of its limitations, but is still considered valuable by some. In this test, carbon dioxide is put through the cervix into the uterus and tubes under pressure. If the tubes are open, the carbon dioxide will pass through the tubes into the abdominal cavity where it is absorbed by the body. The doctor can hear the gas bubbling through the tubes with a stethoscope. If the carbon dioxide does indeed pass through one or both tubes, you will feel some pain in your shoulder joints (of all places) when you sit up. The gas rises and puts pressure on your diaphragm (the muscular membrane wall that separates your abdominal cavity from your lungs and heart). This causes pain which is referred to the shoulder joints. This pain will go away in a few hours when your body absorbs the carbon dioxide. If the gas did not pass through, even under higher pressure, then the diagnosis is still uncertain because it could indicate either scar tissue blockage or tubal spasm.

There is a another procedure called hydrotubation in which a sterile saline solution is injected up through the cervix in a sterile manner with low pressure. The saline solution will flow out through the tubes and into the abdominal cavity, just like the carbon dioxide, if there is no blockage. If all the saline reaches the abdominal cavity, then at least one tube is open. If part of the premeasured saline goes through (does not come back out), there may be a partial blockage, one blocked tube, or spasm of the tube(s). If all of the saline that was put in flows back out, there is a total blockage or a strong spasm of both tubes.

Neither the Rubin test or hydrotubation can show the true nature or position of a blockage, but they are simple and inexpensive, and can sometimes "rinse out" or "blow out" loose debris from the tubes, thus serving a therapeutic purpose.

The main test of fallopian tube patency (openness) is called a *hysterosalpingogram*, which means an X-ray of the uterus (hystero) and tubes (salpinges). In this test, the uterus and tubes are filled with a radio-opaque dye and then X-rayed. You usually receive four to eight X-rays. Modern specialists will try to keep the X-rays down to about four, with some fluoroscopy to locate everything before shooting the pictures.

A hysterosalpingogram is done in an X-ray facility

on an outpatient basis. It provides a lot more information than the simpler office tests, and is considered by most fertility doctors to be essential to a diagnosis. It will clearly show the shape and condition of the uterus and tubes, any malformations, adhesions, and the exact location and degree of scarring. This test can also be therapeutic through a more controlled "flushing out" of the tubes (if the blockage is movable). The dye itself is usually water soluble and easily absorbed by the body. This test will cost over $100.

If you don't want the X-rays and fluoroscopy, you could request the hydrotubation procedure and let your doctor know that you understand and accept its limitations, and the significant limitations of a fertility workup without X-rays.

If the X-rays show that the tubes *are* closed off, the only treatment is surgery. First, your doctor would perform a laparoscopy to see if the tubes are really blocked, the extent of scarring, if tubal surgery is appropriate, etc. For the laparoscopy, he/she makes a small incision in the abdomen to insert the laparoscope, a lighted, optical instrument that enables him to see the ovaries and tubes. Sometimes he might be able to fix something during this procedure, or he may need to move things around a little to see better. In either case, he would make another small incision for instruments. A laparoscopy costs around $700 including hospital fees. You and your doctor would then decide about tubal surgery.

Tubal microsurgery has come a long way in the last few years, and is often successful depending on the location and severity of the occlusion. If you were considering surgery, your doctor would be able to give you ballpark odds on your chances for conception based on your personal condition. This type of surgery is expensive. It usually costs $5000-$7000.

SPERM COUNT

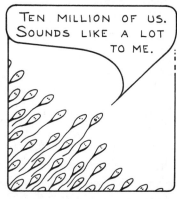

TEN MILLION OF US. SOUNDS LIKE A LOT TO ME.

Sometimes sperm are low in numbers. It only takes one sperm to fertilize an egg, but the sperm have a long and arduous journey to get there. Large numbers are simply killed by the ordinary acid environment of the vagina before they can reach the sperm-sustaining alkaline mucus of the cervix. The cave-like crypts of the cervix, which make the fertility-enhancing mucus, act as a sort of half-way house for the sperm, feeding and housing them on their journey. Once in the uterus, many more of the sperm never find the two holes which lead out of the uterus to the two tubes. Many sperm will swim their tiny lives out, never finding the right door.

Of those that do find the two exits high in the womb, a good many will go up the wrong tube. The egg is only coming down one tube each cycle. These sperm are lost for any practical purposes unless we have the rare event of fraternal twins eggs traveling down separate tubes (both ovulating from the same hormonal stimulus, minutes or hours apart). So you can see why it usually takes a large number of sperm to give you good odds for conception.

A so-called normal sperm count, providing ordinary male fertility, is around 30-60 million sperm per milliliter. These sperm must also have good mobility and motility (many active after a few hours) and morphology (normal size and shape).

Sperm production can be low because of a congenital malformation of the testes, an acute or chronic illness (or its treatment), hormonal deficiencies of the pituitary or thyroid glands, some antibiotics, mumps, nutritional deficiencies (especially protein and vitamins), or exposure to harmful chemicals or radiation.

Sperm counts have been declining in recent years due to environmental pollutants, pesticides, industrial chemicals, etc. The testes are extremely sensitive to these assaults. If the sperm count is marginal or low, it would be wise to conduct the hormone tests, correct poor nutrition, take a good vitamin/mineral supplement, avoid fatigue, and eliminate exposure to industrial chemicals or any form of radiation, at work or at home.

Another factor that can cause a poor showing in the sperm department is local heat around the testes. Even the normal body temperature of 98.6° is too hot. That is why the testicles are suspended away from the body in the scrotum. On a cold day, the scrotum will shrink and hold the testicles close to the body for warmth; on a hot day the scrotum will, if free to do so, hang lower, moving the heat sensitive sperm farther from the body. If a man takes many hot baths or wears tight underwear which holds the scrotum close to the body, or regularly sits on a warm seat of a front engine truck, he can seriously impair his sperm production.

When any of these factors are corrected, it can take up to three months for the sperm count to improve (if it's going to). If the first sperm count is low, ask for another after several months. It may have been a temporary problem.

But even if the sperm count is low there is always a chance for that lone hearty dedicated sperm to make the trip against the odds. Even with a count of, say 10-20 million, your miracle might happen. Where there are any sperm at all, there is hope.

POST-PILL AMENORRHEA

After discontinuing oral contraceptives, some women do not resume their normal cycles and periods for a while. This is more often true of women who had long or irregular cycles before they took the pill. This problem will usually resolve itself in time, but your doctor may want to treat the condition. After discontinuing pills (and for that matter, while on them), you should take a good multivitamin-mineral supplement. Oral contraceptives use up more of certain vitamins and minerals. Be sure the supplement contains vitamin B6, folic acid, and zinc. It is not a good idea to try to conceive right after going off oral contraceptives because the additional hormones of the pill could affect a new fetus. It is best to use another form of birth control for about 6 months before trying to conceive.

INCOMPATIBLE MUCUS

Incompatible mucus from the cervix can occasionally destroy sperm. Some women have an immune response to their husband's sperm. They produce antibodies against the sperm, and this can make conception difficult if not impossible. This condition can be suspected or ruled out by a simple test in the doctor's office called a "post-coital test." The cervical mucus is examined under a microscope, around the time of ovulation, within a few hours after intercourse. The sperm will either be thriving in the mucus, or they will be showing casualties.

HORMONAL IMBALANCE

Hormonal imbalance can cause a lack of ovulation or problems with sustaining conception. There can be a problem with the ovary which secretes the reproductive hormones estrogen and progesterone; or the pituitary gland, which produces the hormones LH—Luteinizing Hormone and FSH—Follicle Stimulating Hormone.

If the pituitary gland does not produce enough FSH to attain critical blood levels, ovulation will be delayed or never occur. There may be a problem with the pituitary itself, or it may not be receiving the signal from the hypothalamus to secrete FSH. The hypothalamus starts the hormonal interplay, and it can be affected by organic or stress-related factors.

If the corpus luteum of the ovary does not secrete enough progesterone, or does not remain active for the required minimum of eleven days, it will not prevent menstruation even if conception has occurred. The embryo needs this time to implant and produce its own menstruation-suppressing hormones. The result is early, often repeated and unnoticed, miscarriage. The basal temperature chart will reveal much about the duration of the corpus luteum function and is helpful in diagnosing this *luteal phase defect* (as it is known).

Sometimes a luteal phase defect is subtle and does not show up on the BBT test. If the charts look fine, sperm are fine, post-coital test is fine, etc., your doctor may want to perform an *endometrial biopsy* to "date the endometrium," and see if the lining is growing as it should under the stimulus of enough progesterone. A small piece of the endometrium is clipped with a special instrument right before the period is due (according to BBT) and sent to a lab. The lab checks to see if the endometrium is thick enough to be about due for menstruation. They estimate the day of the cycle from which it was taken. If the sample is thin and looks like it came from early in the cycle, there is not enough progesterone.

This condition is sometimes treated with progesterone, but it must be pure organic progesterone (in oil) because synthetic progesterone can cause masculinization of a female fetus.

Progesterone of any kind is not approved by the FDA for use in the first trimester of pregnancy. We really don't know the long-term effects of prescribing any hormones or drugs in the first trimester. It is best for pregnant women to avoid all unnecessary drugs.

The pure organic progesterone cannot be taken orally. It is in an oil base and must be injected daily for the duration of the luteal phase. The shots can be rather painful because of the oil base. It can be made up special in vaginal suppository form, but this is not commercially available.

Sometimes a luteal phase defect is treated with an estrogen-like drug (Clomid) to create a "stronger" ovulation, but this can sometimes cause cystic ovaries or multiple births (and perhaps other unforeseen developments). You would want to discuss the options of treatment thoroughly with your doctor.

The inappropriate secretion of the hormone *prolactin* can cause infertility through suppression of ovulation. Prolactin is another hormone produced by the anterior pituitary gland. It is usually released only during lactation in response to the baby's nursing. It stimulates the production of milk and suppresses ovulation. In a few women, the pituitary secretes high levels of prolactin, sometimes from benign prolactin-producing tumor(s) of the pituitary. High prolactin levels will usually cause a milk secretion from the breasts in a non-lactating woman, and a lack of periods (amenorrhea). This condition can be diagnosed by hormone tests and treated with drugs or occasionally surgery. Incidentally, any secretion from non-nursing breasts should be checked right away by a doctor.

Another endocrine gland, the thyroid gland, can be underactive and cause infertility. Your doctor might give you a blood test to measure the thyroid hormone. If it is low, a thyroid supplement would probably be prescribed, and might improve fertility.

ANOVULATORY CYCLES

If it is observed from the BBT test that the basal temperature does not rise in the second phase of the cycle, it is called a "monophasic cycle." Most monophasic cycles are anovulatory—without ovulation. Occasionally, a woman is ovulating normally, and her corpus luteum is producing plenty of progesterone each cycle, but her body does not react to the thermal effects of progesterone and her temperature does not rise. This situation can only be detected by blood hormone tests for progesterone in the second part of the cycle, or an endometrial biopsy performed just a few days before the period.

If the cycles are truly anovulatory, your doctor may want to try to stimulate ovulation with hormones. There can be short-term complications of hormone therapy through overstimulation of the ovaries, and possibly unknown long-term effects.

AMENORRHEA

Amenorrhea means no periods with no ovulation. There is *primary amenorrhea* where the periods never started during puberty, and there is *secondary amenorrhea* where you have menstruated in the past but do not now; the cyclic process has begun, but then stops. Primary amenorrhea, if it goes into the very late teens or twenties, might be a glandular problem and needs medical investigation. But many athletic and thin girls don't get their periods until they are older because to go into this phase of puberty requires a minimum level of body fat, a certain proportion of fat to total weight. It's hard for some teenage runners or dancers, swimmers, etc., to keep any fat on their bodies. (Conversely, some plump girls can get their periods at a younger than average age.)

It is not uncommon for a woman to experience

temporary amenorrhea when she moves—changes location, home, friends, etc. Remember, the first signal for the whole thing to begin is from the hypothalamus, and the hypothalamus is sensitive to any kind of stress or change. Sometimes going away to school will cause temporary amenorrhea. Long work hours or a stressful job can interfere with ovulation. Family problems can cause delayed or irregular ovulation. Some medications can cause suppression of ovulation, as can illness, under-nourishment, partial starvation (from extreme dieting, fad diets, fasting) and obesity.

If your amenorrhea has been prolonged, your doctor will want to run some hormone level tests to rule out more physiological problems of the pituitary, such as benign tumors, high prolactin levels, etc.

For the woman who goes long periods of time without ovulation, there is also a risk of overgrowth of the lining of the womb from prolonged unopposed estrogen stimulation of the womb, possibly even cancer in certain cases. Endometrial biopsy is important to detect any abnormal endometrial cells early.

If the tests prove OK and there just isn't any cyclic action, then it is up to you, with the consultation of your doctor, to decide whether to embark on hormone treatments for this condition or just wait and try to remove any physical and mental stress from your life. Many women need only wait and their periods will return. If you decide to wait, you should have the endometrial biopsies performed on a regular schedule.

INADEQUATE CERVICAL MUCUS

Inadequate cervical mucus or inflammation of the cervix can make conception difficult. (More about cervical mucus later.) The fertile cervical mucus is important to the sperm. Sometimes infection, inflammation, hormone deficiency or cauterization of the cervix can cause a deficiency of this special fertile fluid and a lowering of fecundity. Cervicitis should be treated, as should chronic or periodic yeast infections which can thicken the mucus or make intercourse painful.

ENDOMETRIOSIS

Endometriosis can cause infertility. This is a special condition wherein some of the uterine lining tissue ends up outside the uterus in the abdominal cavity. Then, every month, when the uterine lining builds up to nourish and sustain a potential embryo, it also builds up from the displaced tissue outside the womb. This can cause pain and may cause adhesions which can interfere with the proper transport of the egg through the tube. If pregnancy can be achieved, it will help this condition by stopping the cyclic build-up of the endometrium. If you have endometriosis, your doctor may want to do a laparoscopy to assess the situation and decide on a course of treatment.

DIETARY DEFICIENCIES

Dietary deficiencies can interfere with fertility. Too little protein can cause irregular or absent ovulation as can extreme thinness and fad diets with their accompanying general nutritional deficiencies. Obesity can also be a factor in infertility, whether caused by overeating or an underactive thyroid.

AGE AND FERTILITY

Age itself can contribute to infertility. There is a general decline in female fertility that begins in the third decade. Women in their thirties and forties are usually less fertile than women in their twenties. Some of this decline is probably caused by a longer exposure to life's fertility limiters such as infection, endometriosis, poor diet, etc.

In any woman, an embryo sometimes fails to implant properly or gets off to a wrong start in early cell divison, and is lost in the normal menstrual period or a "late" period. Older women may have a somewhat lower rate of implantation due to a generally older reproductive system.

Also, for about five years preceeding menopause, some of the cycles can become very long or very short, with increasing numbers of anovulatory cycles, with or without periods. These years can still be fertile, although less so than before.

YOUR BASAL
TEMPERATURE

THE BASAL TEMPERATURE
CAN HELP DETERMINE
IF AND WHEN YOU OVULATE.

How and why can it do this? A hormone in the female menstrual cycle called progesterone causes the basal temperature (body at rest temperature) to rise by about 1/2 of a degree Fahrenheit. This hormone is not significantly released into the bloodstream until after ovulation. So a basal temperature that is higher later in the cycle than it was earlier in the cycle is evidence of probable ovulation.

Temperatures in the early part of the cycle will be relatively low.

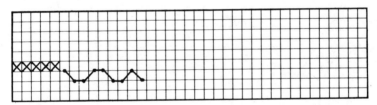

When ovulation has happened and progesterone enters the picture, the temperature rises.

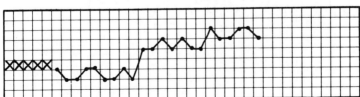

37

To keep track of the thermal changes in your cycle, you can take your basal temperature first thing each morning and record it on a chart and connect each dot with a line. You should get a curve that begins low in the early part of the cycle and rises at, or right after, ovulation, remaining high until your following period.

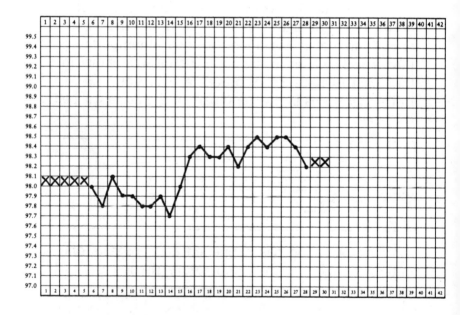

WE CANNOT TELL EXACTLY WHEN OVULATION OCCURS. We can tell when it seems to be approaching by a build-up and liquefying of the cervical mucus (more on this later). We can tell when ovulation has passed by the higher temperatures. We can only gather presumptive evidence of ovulation and place the event within a day or two between the "before" and "after" signs.

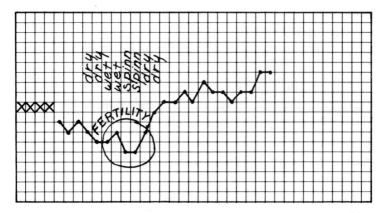

These days during which ovulation is probably occurring are the optimum days for intercourse. The only way we could know the exact moment or even the exact day of ovulation would be to be in there with a laparoscope* watching. So we have to establish our signs of ovulation and do the best we can within two or three days on either side.

*Laparoscope: a lighted optical surgical device [FOR LOOKING IN LAPS?]

RECORDING YOUR BASAL TEMPERATURE

On the basal temperature charts, you will find the "day of the cycle" printed across the top of the squares **(A)**. *The first day of your period is the first day of the cycle.* The second day of your period is "day 2" on the chart, etc.

Above the "days of the cycle," you will find the "day of the week" **(B)**. You should fill in the days of the week, starting with the first day of your period/cycle. If it was Wednesday, put a "W" in the slot and fill in all the days of the week.

Then, fill in the dates in the slots for "day of the month." If "day 1" of the cycle was August 14, put a "14" in the first slot, and continue with the dates **(C)**.

Start taking your temperature on "day 6" of your cycle unless you sometimes have very short cycles (under 25 days), then start earlier. Locate the temperature readings on the left side of the chart. If your temp was 97.9° **(a)**, follow the line next to 97.9° across the page until you come to the column of "day 6" (M, Aug 19). On the center of the line, under, "day 6," place a dot **(b)**. Do the same for the following days. Connect the dots with lines. If you skip a day of your temperature, make a dotted line **(c)**.

Basal Temperature Chart

Chart number_____

Name _____ Shortest Previous Cycle_____

Month(s) _____ Longest Previous Cycle_____

Year_____ Length of this cycle_____

(C)

Day of

month | 14 15 16 17 18 19 20 21 22 23 24 25 26 27 28 29 30 31 1 2 3 4 5 6 7 8 9 10 11

week | W T F S S M T W T F S S M T W T F S S M T W T F S S M T W

(B)

(A)

Temperature

| 99.5 | 99.4 | 99.3 | 99.2 | 99.1 | 99.0 | 98.9 | 98.8 | 98.7 | 98.6 | 98.5 | 98.4 | 98.3 | 98.2 | 98.1 | 98.0 | 97.9 | 97.8 | 97.7 | 97.6 | 97.5 | 97.4 | 97.3 | 97.2 | 97.1 | 97.0 |

(b)

(c)

(a)

Mucus, other observations and disturbances

UNDERSTANDING YOUR TEMPERATURE CHART

YOU WILL HAVE RELATIVELY LOW TEMPERATURES FROM THE TIME OF YOUR PERIOD UNTIL YOU OVULATE. OVULATION WILL CAUSE A RISE OF ABOUT 6/10 OF ONE DEGREE (SIX LINES ON YOUR CHART). THIS RISE CAN HAPPEN IN A DAY OR IT CAN STAIR-STEP UP OVER A PERIOD OF SEVERAL DAYS.

Ovulation took place right before the rise in temperature or anywhere during the rise from low to high.

You may not have such a drastic rise, but if the temperatures late in the cycle are generally higher than those early in the cycle, then you are ovulating.

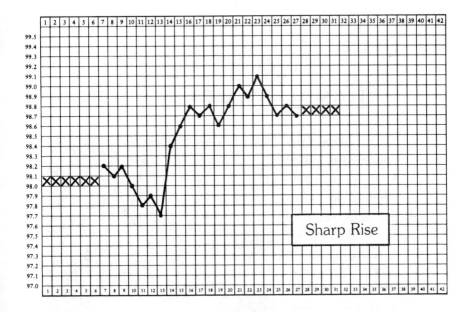

Sharp Rise

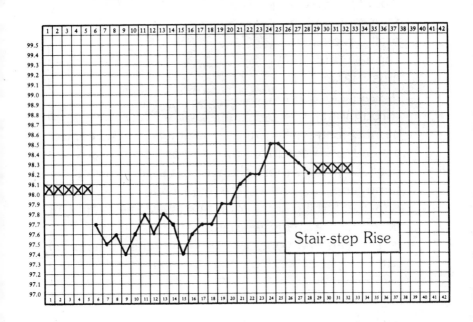

Stair-step Rise

TAKING YOUR BASAL TEMPERATURE

The basal temperature is taken first thing upon awakening, while the body is still at its "basal level." It is important to take your temperature before getting up, eating, drinking, smoking, etc. You can take your temp orally, rectally or vaginally but you must take it in the same location throughout the 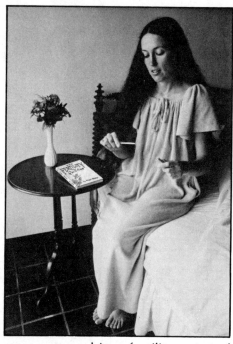 month. Later, if you are seeking fertility control instead of pregnancy, oral temps are not advised because there is more chance for a slightly inaccurate temp and the stakes are high. But now, for this personal fertility study, oral temps are fine and might be easier for many women.

You can find your basal body temperature (BBT) with a special kind of thermometer called a basal thermometer.

HOW TO READ
YOUR THERMOMETER

To read your temperature on your thermometer, hold it near a good light and turn it slowly until you can see a shiny silver line (mercury) that goes from the silver bulb part way out into the numbers and lines.

BASAL THERMOMETER

A basal thermometer is different from a regular fever thermometer because it records just the degrees of 95° to 100° and has a mark for each 1/10th of a degree.

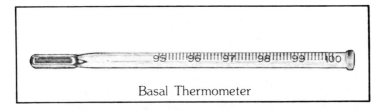

Basal Thermometer

The numbers represent whole degrees and the lines between the numbers represent parts of that whole degree.

Look at the number which the mercury (silver line) has already passed. That is the number of whole degrees. Next, count each small line which the mercury has passed. This number of small lines is the number of 1/10 degrees. You express the 1/10 degrees by saying "point six" for six-tenths (6/10).

You say "point two" for two-tenths (2/10) of a degree. Here are some examples:

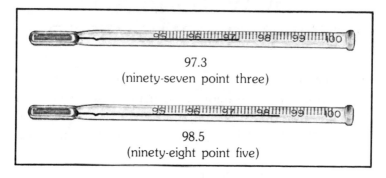

97.3
(ninety-seven point three)

98.5
(ninety-eight point five)

REGULAR THERMOMETER

The fever thermometer only has numbers for every other degree—the even numbers, i.e. 96°, 98°, 100°.

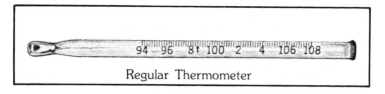

Regular Thermometer

A regular thermometer has more degrees on the glass tube than a basal thermometer, and doesn't have room for each whole number. The odd numbers are shown by a tall line.

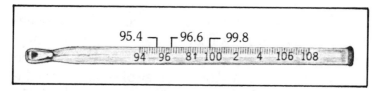

The tall line between 94° and 96° is for 95°. The tall line between 96° and 98° is for 97°. The shorter lines represent two-tenths (2/10) of a degree each.

Count each small line that the mercury has passed as 2/10 of a degree instead of 1/10 of a degree. Count by "twos" for each small line: "point two, point four, point six," etc.

If you use a regular thermometer to chart your basal temperature, you will have to *EITHER:* estimate the halfway points between the short lines (whew!) in order to record each .1 (1/10));

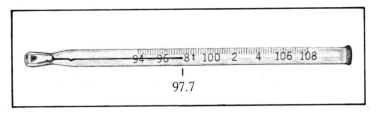

97.7

OR: only record every .2 (2/10) on the chart, i.e., 98.2°, 98.4°, 98.6°, etc. Your chart would look this:

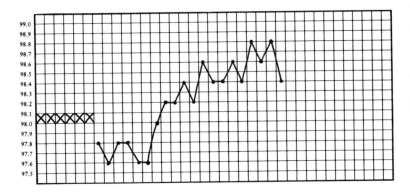

I suggest you invest in a basal thermometer (ask your druggist) because it is easier to read in the wee morning hours and will give you more accuracy to the 1/10 of a degree.

Here are some examples of temperature charts:

This is a very typical biphasic temperature chart. She probably ovulated somewhere between the 13th and the 16th day of this cycle. She had a 30 day cycle with 15 days of elevated temperatures.

Basal Temperature Chart

Chart number_____

Name _____ Shortest Previous Cycle_____

Month(s) _____ Longest Previous Cycle_____

Year_____ Length of this cycle __30__

Day of month

Day of week

Temperature

99.5
99.4
99.3
99.2
99.1
99.0
98.9
98.8
98.7
98.6
98.5
98.4
98.3
98.2
98.1
98.0
97.9
97.8
97.7
97.6
97.5
97.4
97.3
97.2
97.1
97.0

PERIOD

Mucus, other observations and disturbances

Here is another typical temperature chart. She ovulated a little earlier than most (probably around day 11-13) and, consequently, has a slightly short cycle of 26 days. She had 13 days of higher temperatures. (Don't count the temperature of the day she got her next period.)

If it is unclear which day the higher temperatures started, average all temps from the cycle. Those temps at or above the "average" temp are the highs.

Basal Temperature Chart

Chart number_____

Name _____ Shortest Previous Cycle_____

Month(s) _____ Longest Previous Cycle_____

Year_____ Length of this cycle 26

Day of																																											
month																																											
week																																											

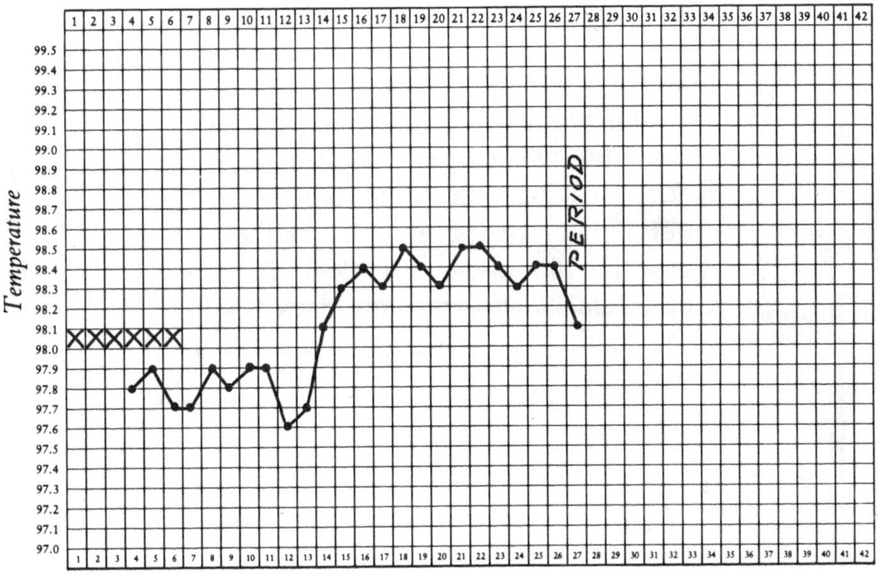

Mucus, other observations and disturbances

This woman has long cycles of 35-42 days. In this cycle, she ovulated around the 23rd-25th day and had a period about two weeks later. If she thought that the 14th day was fertile for her, she could easily miss the few days around the 24th day when she was really ovulating.

Basal Temperature Chart

Chart number_____

Name _____

Month(s) _____

Year_____

Shortest Previous Cycle_____

Longest Previous Cycle_____

Length of this cycle _39_

Day of | month | week

Temperature

99.5 99.4 99.3 99.2 99.1 99.0 98.9 98.8 98.7 98.6 98.5 98.4 98.3 98.2 98.1 98.0 97.9 97.8 97.7 97.6 97.5 97.4 97.3 97.2 97.1 97.0

Mucus, other observations and disturbances

This woman has short cycles, and hence, early ovulation. This cycle was only 21 days long, but may be normal since she had 12 days of elevated temperatures. (Many women have a short cycle like this occasionally, maybe every year or two.) Because she usually has short cycles, she takes her temperature during her period to see which temps are low, and how low. If she was counting on "day 14" being her fertile time, she would miss her ovulation which took place around day 8 or 9. By "day 14," the egg would be long gone.

Basal Temperature Chart

Chart number _____

Name _____ Shortest Previous Cycle _____

Month(s) _____ Longest Previous Cycle _____

Year _____ Length of this cycle _21_

Day of month / week

| | 1 | 2 | 3 | 4 | 5 | 6 | 7 | 8 | 9 | 10 | 11 | 12 | 13 | 14 | 15 | 16 | 17 | 18 | 19 | 20 | 21 | 22 | 23 | 24 | 25 | 26 | 27 | 28 | 29 | 30 | 31 | 32 | 33 | 34 | 35 | 36 | 37 | 38 | 39 | 40 | 41 | 42 |

Temperature

99.5
99.4
99.3
99.2
99.1
99.0
98.9
98.8
98.7
98.6
98.5
98.4
98.3
98.2
98.1
98.0
97.9
97.8
97.7
97.6
97.5
97.4
97.3
97.2
97.1
97.0

Mucus, other observations and disturbances

Here is an "anovulatory" cycle. This woman did not ovulate in this cycle. Her temperature chart did not show a "biphasic curve" with the early temperatures lower than the later temperatures. There is no evidence of ovulation on this chart even though there was an apparently normal period starting on the 30th day. You can tell that there was no ovulation because the temperature did not rise.

Basal Temperature Chart

Chart number_____

Name _____ Shortest Previous Cycle_____

Month(s) _____ Longest Previous Cycle____

Year_____   Length of this cycle *29*

Day of
month
week

| 1 | 2 | 3 | 4 | 5 | 6 | 7 | 8 | 9 | 10 | 11 | 12 | 13 | 14 | 15 | 16 | 17 | 18 | 19 | 20 | 21 | 22 | 23 | 24 | 25 | 26 | 27 | 28 | 29 | 30 | 31 | 32 | 33 | 34 | 35 | 36 | 37 | 38 | 39 | 40 | 41 | 42 |

Temperature

99.5
99.4
99.3
99.2
99.1
99.0
98.9
98.8
98.7
98.6
98.5
98.4
98.3
98.2
98.1
98.0
97.9
97.8
97.7
97.6
97.5
97.4
97.3
97.2
97.1
97.0

Mucus, other observations and disturbances

This woman had a rise in temperature but it didn't stay up for the usual 12-16 days. Her temperature only remained elevated for 6 days in this cycle, This is likely a factor in her subfertility. (But sometimes short-cycled women have relatively short high-temp phases of 10 or 11 days and are quite fertile.)

Basal Temperature Chart

Name _____ Shortest Previous Cycle_____

Month(s) _____ Longest Previous Cycle_____

Year_____ Length of this cycle **24**

Day of month

week

Temperature

99.5
99.4
99.3
99.2
99.1
99.0
98.9
98.8
98.7
98.6
98.5
98.4
98.3
98.2
98.1
98.0
97.9
97.8
97.7
97.6
97.5
97.4
97.3
97.2
97.1
97.0

PERIOD

Mucus, other observations and disturbances

At first glance, you might think this was an anovulatory cycle because all the temperatures are about the same and there isn't a half-a-degree difference between the early and the late temperatures. But if you were to draw a line across the highest of the early low temps, you would see that the later temps are indeed higher.

Basal Temperature Chart

Chart number_____

Name _____ Shortest Previous Cycle_____

Month(s) _____ Longest Previous Cycle_____

Year_____ Length of this cycle _31_

Day of month | week

Temperature

99.5
99.4
99.3
99.2
99.1
99.0
98.9
98.8
98.7
98.6
98.5
98.4
98.3
98.2
98.1
98.0
97.9
97.8
97.7
97.6
97.5
97.4
97.3
97.2
97.1
97.0

Mucus, other observations and disturbances

Her temperature was pretty erratic during the first phase of the cycle. But except for a couple of early high oddballs, the later temps were higher than the earlier ones. She probably ovulated right before or during the final climb, between days 13 and 16.

Basal Temperature Chart

Chart number_____

Name _____ Shortest Previous Cycle_____

Month(s) _____ Longest Previous Cycle_____

Year_____ Length of this cycle **28**

Day of | month | | | | | | | | | | | | | | | | | | | | | | | | | | | | | | | | | | | | | | | | |
| week | | | | | | | | | | | | | | | | | | | | | | | | | | | | | | | | | | | | | | | | |

Temperature

| | 1 | 2 | 3 | 4 | 5 | 6 | 7 | 8 | 9 | 10 | 11 | 12 | 13 | 14 | 15 | 16 | 17 | 18 | 19 | 20 | 21 | 22 | 23 | 24 | 25 | 26 | 27 | 28 | 29 | 30 | 31 | 32 | 33 | 34 | 35 | 36 | 37 | 38 | 39 | 40 | 41 | 42 |

99.5
99.4
99.3
99.2
99.1
99.0
98.9
98.8
98.7
98.6
98.5
98.4
98.3
98.2
98.1
98.0
97.9
97.8
97.7
97.6
97.5
97.4
97.3
97.2
97.1
97.0

PERIOD

Mucus, other observations and disturbances

This woman probably had a fever early in her cycle. She noted her illness on her chart. The fever temperatures were higher than her usual late cycle "highs." Sometimes a cold or a sore throat can raise your temp a few tenths (rather than several whole degrees). So note any illness on your chart.

Basal Temperature Chart

Chart number_____

Name _____ Shortest Previous Cycle_____

Month(s) _____ Longest Previous Cycle_____

Year_____ Length of this cycle **34**

Day of month / week

Temperature

99.5 99.4 99.3 99.2 99.1 99.0 98.9 98.8 98.7 98.6 98.5 98.4 98.3 98.2 98.1 98.0 97.9 97.8 97.7 97.6 97.5 97.4 97.3 97.2 97.1 97.0

PERIOD

Mucus, other observations and disturbances

flu flu flu well well well

This woman got pregnant this month. Do you see anything unusual about her chart? Count the days of high temps. If pregnancy should occur, the temperature will remain elevated past the lifespan of the corpus luteum—which is 12 to 16 days, remember? In fact, 20 days of elevated temperature is almost certainly proof of pregnancy.

Basal Temperature Chart

Chart number_____

Name _____ Shortest Previous Cycle_____

Month(s) _____ Longest Previous Cycle_____

Year_____ Length of this cycle_____

Day of month / week

Temperature

| | 1 | 2 | 3 | 4 | 5 | 6 | 7 | 8 | 9 | 10 | 11 | 12 | 13 | 14 | 15 | 16 | 17 | 18 | 19 | 20 | 21 | 22 | 23 | 24 | 25 | 26 | 27 | 28 | 29 | 30 | 31 | 32 | 33 | 34 | 35 | 36 | 37 | 38 | 39 | 40 | 41 | 42 |

99.5, 99.4, 99.3, 99.2, 99.1, 99.0, 98.9, 98.8, 98.7, 98.6, 98.5, 98.4, 98.3, 98.2, 98.1, 98.0, 97.9, 97.8, 97.7, 97.6, 97.5, 97.4, 97.3, 97.2, 97.1, 97.0

Mucus, other observations and disturbances

INFREQUENT OVULATION WITH PERIODS

You may see from your charts that although you have pretty regular periods, you only seem to ovulate every few months. If you didn't take your temperature, you might never know this.

It is very possible to ovulate infrequently and have a period every 26-35 days. These anovulatory "periods" are usually pretty light and uncomplicated (if you ever took "the Pill," you might recognize them as similar to "pill periods": short, easy, few or no cramps). Anovulatory periods are usually light because they only consist of the estrogen-induced build-up of the lining of the womb. The endometrium goes through more of its preparation and proliferation after the release of progesterone from the corpus luteum. But if there is no ovulation, there is no corpus luteum and no progesterone. You still might shed an estrogen-induced lining approximately monthly. Your chart would look something like this:

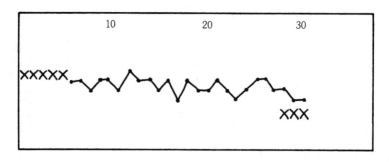

The next cycle could be ovulatory, your chart would look more like this:

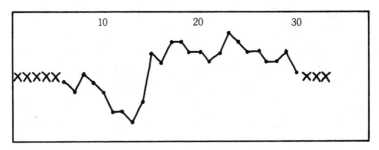

Maybe only every second or third cycle looks ovulatory from the charts. This means that you can probably only conceive for about four days every 60-90 days. Well, if you knew this was happening, you could pay special attention to your mucus and you might feel more patient with your situation. You would know that (if all else is working right) it is probably just a matter of time.

Some women may go 60-90 days with no period. In such a case, it's not that you're really "missing" periods. If you only menstruate every 90 days, you are not "missing" two out of three periods; but it is taking about 75 days for your hormones to reach their critical levels for ovulation to occur. The chart would look something like this:

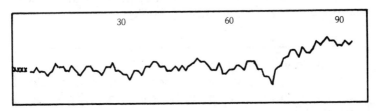

Some women normally have only 4-6 periods a year throughout their reproductive lifetime. Also, long irregular cycles are not really unusual for anyone under twenty-five. It is sometimes characteristic of the young, still-developing reproductive system for the cycles to be long. Also, many girls and young women have unusually short cycles in the first few years of their female cycles. Fifty-day cycles and twenty-one day cycles are both "normal" for many young women in this age group.

By the time a woman is in her mid-twenties, she is likely to have the more usual 26-35 day cycle length, although some will naturally have the very short or very long cycles through maturity. According to Dr. Rudolph Vollman, an international authority on the menstrual cycle, it takes 10 years past menarche (1st period) for a young woman's reproductive system to fully develop and mature. So if your periods commenced at age 14, your system is not finished developing until you are about 24.

Long or irregular cycles can also be caused by physical, mental, or emotional stress. Many things can delay ovulation or even stop it for a long time.

In the mature woman, long, long cycles with their accompanying rare ovulation may just be a genetic trait. If this is your tendency, ask your female relatives if they have similar cycles.

Women with a long pre-ovulatory phase are at risk to develop an overstimulated endometrium, and should arrange with their doctors to have endometrial biopsies occasionally.

CERVICAL MUCUS
AN INDICATOR OF OVULATION

The cyclic changes in your cervical mucus can be helpful in ovulation detection. This mucus is found at the opening of the vagina. It can be thick or thin, white, yellow or clear, scant or abundant according to hormonal changes.

You are creating cervical mucus all the time. It is produced by special cells up inside the cervix and changes character during the monthly cycle. You may have noticed this normal discharge and wondered why it was profuse at times and absent at other times.

There are about 100 gland-like crypts producing cervical mucus.

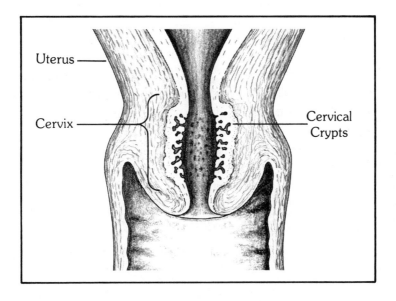

In the beginning and end of the cycle, when the hormone estrogen is low, the mucus is scant, sticky and opaque with cellular matter. In the middle of the cycle, it changes to fertile type mucus. As the estrogen level increases, preparing for ovulation, the quantity of mucus increases. It becomes thinner and milkier. Then with still more estrogen, it gets clearer and more watery. At the estrogen peak, right before ovulation, it gets slick and glassy and you may be able to stretch an unbroken shimmering thread of it between your thumb and forefinger or between two slides. This condition is known by the German term *Spinnbarkeit*, or *Spinn* for short.

At this fertile time, the mucus has usually increased to ten times what it was earlier. The abundant fertile mucus is very helpful to sperm. It nourishes them, guides them upward through its fiber-like channels, and protects them from the acid pH of your vagina (the mucus is alkaline).

After ovulation, the hormone progesterone causes the mucus to change to the sticky, infertile type within a day or two. Progesterone inhibits the mucus producing cells of the cervix and the mucus again becomes scant, thick, sticky, and opaque white or yellow from cellular matter and protein content. Infertile mucus, aside from indicating that you are not ovulating right now, also forms a thick criss-cross barrier across the cervix and keeps sperm and anything else from getting past the cervix into the womb for most of the cycle.

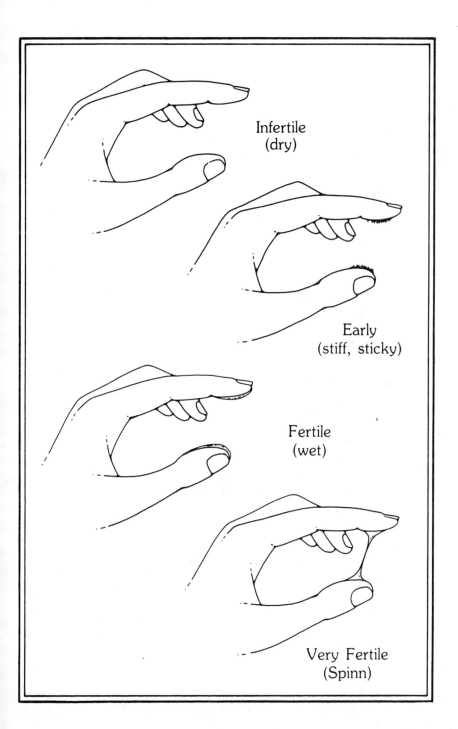

Infertile
(dry)

Early
(stiff, sticky)

Fertile
(wet)

Very Fertile
(Spinn)

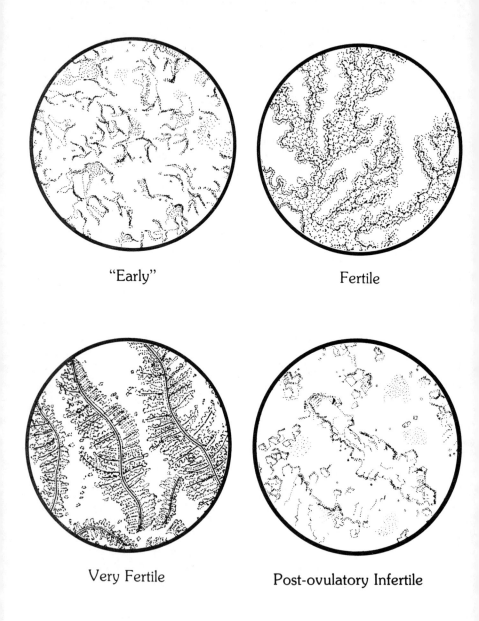

"Early"

Fertile

Very Fertile

Post-ovulatory Infertile

The wet, fertile mucus is also noted by its ability to "fern," that is to form fern-like patterns when it is dried on a slide. If you have a microscope, you could look at it. This ferning is caused by a higher salt content during the height of the mucus production.

There is usually a substantial increase in mucus from dry to sticky to creamy, to wet or Spinn. But the quality is more important than the quantity. Some women never see Spinn, but notice the increase in wetness. Some women have their wet mucus increasing over 4-5 days, and culminating with lots of clear, slippery Spinn. Others build up only a small amount of milky wetness over a few days and then dry up after ovulation. You will come to recognize your own pattern.

If you do get Spinn or lots of wetness, it is an ideal time to make love. The last day of the wettest or Spinn-type mucus is the most fertile day of the cycle and is usually either the day of or the day before ovulation. The day before ovulation is very fertile because you can make love on this day and have the sperm in there ready and waiting for the egg to emerge.

Any mucus means ovulation may be approaching.

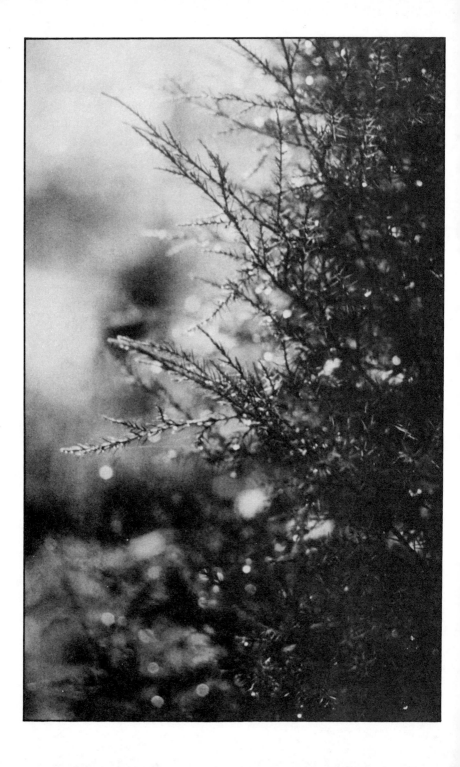

Q & A

Q: My temperature stays low for about 50 days, then it only gets higher for 12 days. Am I ovulating?

A: Probably. You sometimes have long cycles of 60 days. It is taking a long time for your follicles to get enough hormone stimulus to ovulate, about 50 days. But if your temperature did eventually go up, then you are ovulating and, all other things normal, you could conceive. You can see that in a 50 or 60 day cycle, it would be easy to miss making love at ovulation. Watch your mucus for signs of approaching fertility.

Q: One cycle, my temperature rose and two other months, it didn't. What is happening?

A: If this happens regularly, you might only be ovulating every few months. It will be more difficult to conceive, but hopefully not impossible.

Q: I have lots of fertile-looking mucus late in my cycle, after ovulation seems to be over. It starts about a week to 10 days past my ovulation mucus. Am I possibly ovulating twice?

A: No, you are not ovulating twice in one cycle,

unless it is within a few hours with fraternal twins. That fertile-looking mucus late in your cycle is a result of hormone changes leading to your period. Your BBT may also fall right before your period. The hormone that keeps your BBT high and your mucus scant starts to fade a day or two before your period.

Q: My temperature jumps around quite a bit in the first part of my cycle, before ovulation. Once I ovulate, it gets high and stays there, but I wondered about that first part.

A: It's quite all right for your temperature to be a little wild in the early segment of your cycle. Some women's temperatures stay low at this time and some jump around. But you will find that in general, the temperatures before ovulation are lower than those after ovulation.

Q: I get a lot of mucus before I make love when I've been dry all day. Is this fertile mucus?

A: It may be fertile mucus from your cervix or it may be from the lubricating glands right inside your vagina. If you check your mucus when you are ready to make love, it may be the local lubricating mucus. But if you check before you are even thinking about making love, and it is wet and slippery, it is probably fertile mucus from your cervix. If there is any doubt, go ahead and make love.

Q: I am very regular with my menstrual cycle. Does this mean I am ovulating?

A: You cannot tell by your regularity. You can have a

period every 26-29 days and not ovulate. If you have cramps and a heavy flow, you are more likely to be ovulating. An anovulatory cycle often results in a light, painless period. However, many women who do ovulate have scant periods. The only way to really tell is to keep a basal temperature chart. A biphasic curve (low early, high later) is evidence of probable ovulation. A flat curve usually is indicative of an anovulatory cycle.

Q: My cycles vary a lot in length. The last eight have been: 30 days, 27, 25, 32, 34, 26, 32 and 28 days. Is this a problem?

A: No. It is quite normal for the cycles to vary as yours do. Most women have some variation in their cycle length. The "every 28 days" woman is the exception, not the rule. This has nothing to do with your fertility.

Q: My husband had a sperm count and it was 25 million. Is this a lot?

A: Actually, 25 million is borderline low. Of course, it only takes one, but it is generally considered that around 20 million or below is pretty low. Many of the sperm are killed by the acid condition of the vagina; many never find their way from the uterine cavity to a tube. Still more go up the wrong tube. So, statistically you need to start out with a lot to have very many reach their destination. It is also important whether the sperm are healthy, have good motility, etc. With a moderately low sperm count of otherwise normal looking sperm, it would be beneficial to save up some sperm for the few days that are optimum.

Q: I can't say exactly how long my cycles are because I can't determine which is the first day of my period. I usually have some spotting before the flow actually begins. Is this spotting the first day of my cycle?

A: You can tell if the spotting is the real beginning of your period by checking your basal temperature. If the temperature has started to drop from its elevated phase, then the spotting is the beginning of the period. If the basal temperature remains high during the spotting, and drops the day of the heavier flow, then the day of the increased flow is "day 1" of the cycle (and the period).

Q: If my basal temperature chart looks normal, will I get pregnant?

A: The basal temperature only tells us about your ovulation. It cannot diagnose blocked tubes or a low sperm count, etc. If your ovulation appears normal, you may want to have your doctor test for other factors.

Q: I only have periods about three times a year. Can I get pregnant?

A: If all else is normal, you can probably get pregnant, but it may take some time. You are only able to conceive for 3 or 4 days each cycle and you are only having a few cycles (long ones) per year. Approximately two weeks before each of your periods, you are fertile for a few days. You will need to watch for Spinn mucus and make love at that time. If your temperature rises after some fertile-looking mucus, that was ovulation. If it doesn't rise, keep checking the mucus for another fertile-looking batch and try it again. If you have Spinn, and then make love, and observe an elevated temperature during the same few days, your chances for conception are good. It may not work the first time, so keep watching for mucus, keep recording your temperature, and keep trying.

Q: I have taken my temperature for six cycles and it looks normal for ovulation. What now?

A: If you are clearly ovulating, and your temperature always remains elevated for 12-16 days in the second phase of your cycles, you are not having a fertility problem due to ovulation. You and your doctor will probably want to check for other factors such as scarred tubes or your husband's sperm count.

Q: I have a lot of yeast infections. Can this affect my fertility?

A: Many women become pregnant if they have yeast or other infections. But yeast can be a factor in subfertility for a couple of reasons. First, intercourse can be very painful and unappealing if you have yeast, and so it can cause you to miss your fertile times. Also, the yeast infection can make your mucus curdy, stiff, or otherwise inhospitable to sperm. Get it treated with appropriate vaginal suppositories or cream so you can get over it. If it is chronic, you may need treatment for a full cycle and for several days following your period for the next couple of cycles. Don't make love when you have yeast, as this can spread the colonies and make it worse.

Q: Sometimes when we try to have sex at certain times to coincide with my fertile mucus, my husband seems to become temporarily impotent. What should we do?

A: It is fairly common for men or women to feel the pressure to "perform" if their sex life is not completely spontaneous. If "timing" intercourse is making either of you uncomfortable, you should probably not do it. If you both agree in theory to do it, but it isn't working out, then stop for a while and forget about it. Later, you could try a more informal timing, i.e., try to get some loving in once or twice during the fertile time, but avoid strict rules. Cuddle a lot. Laugh a lot. Maintain your loving attitude and your sense of humor; they are what is most important in the long run.

Q: How do I find a doctor?

A: If you want to have most or all of the tests performed by a doctor, then you should seek out a gynecologist who has infertility as a major part of his/her practice. You would want someone who has the time and interest to invest in continuing education in this field. Sometimes your gynecologist is primarily an obstetrician, who does a little infertility work on the side.

Ask if infertility is a major part of their practice; do they do the more complicated tests and surgery themselves? If your doctor does tubal surgery, and you might need it, ask how many times a year they do it, and what is their success rate. Don't be afraid to shop around for a doctor. If you don't feel comfortable with a doctor, if he/she won't communicate with you well, if you feel you are being pushed to surgery too fast, find another doctor. In matters of surgery it is always best to get a second opinion. You can also call your local medical society for recommendations. Make sure your doctor is board-certified in his/her specialty.

Q: What is DES, and what does it have to do with fertility?

A: DES (Diethylstilbestrol) is a synthetic estrogen that was used in the 1940s and 1950s to prevent miscarriage. (It didn't.) It was given to several million women in their first trimester of pregnancy. It was later proven to cause irregularities of the cervix and sometimes a tendency to cervical cancer in daughters born to these women. Their sons have a high rate of infertility and abnormalities of the testes.

DES daughters can have fertility problems, but not as often as DES sons. If your mother took DES when she was pregnant with you, you will need careful monitoring by a specially-trained gynecologist all of your life. DES sons need to be monitored by a urologist and taught self-examination of the testes, as they are more susceptible to cancer of the testicles than most men. DES-induced cancers of the cervix and the testes are treatable if detected early. For more information on DES, you can contact (and support) DES ACTION/National, Long Island Jewish Hillside Medical Center, New Hyde Park, NY 11040.

Q: Are sperm affected by heat?

A: Yes. Sperm don't even do well at body temperature (98.6°), much less anything higher. The testicles are located outside the body cavity so they can stay a little cooler. For optimum fertility, your mate should avoid hot baths (an ancient form of birth control in the Orient) and tight-fitting underwear that would hold the testicles close to the body. Hot tubs and saunas are out.

Q: How can I tell from my chart when I usually ovulate?

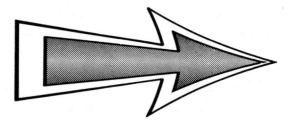

A: You can estimate when ovulation took place on a completed chart. Starting with the last day of the cycle (the day before the next period), count backward eleven days and make a line. Count back five more days and make another line. Ovulation probably took place between the 12th and the 16th day back from the period, (soon before the rise in temperature or anywhere along the rise).

ESTIMATING THE TIME OF
OVULATION
(WITH HINDSIGHT)

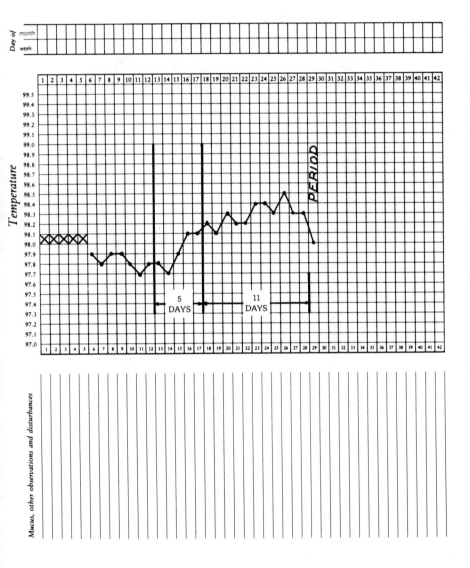

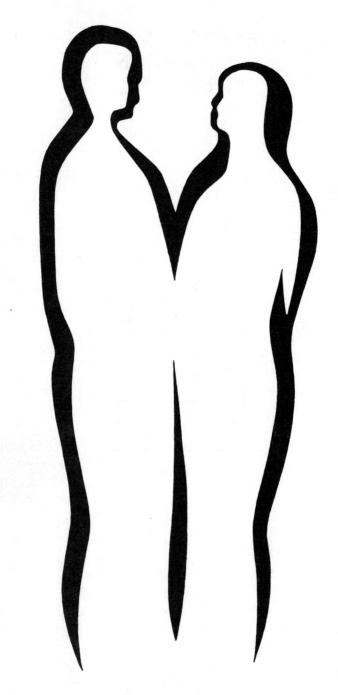

TIMING

You can usually use the temperature chart to establish whether or not you are ovulating and whether or not there is an adequate high temperature phase of at least 10 days—an indication of good hormone levels to sustain a conception. The temperature chart can tell you the approximate pattern of the cycle and to a certain extent, when to expect future ovulation. But the basal temperature chart cannot predict the 1 or 2 days preceeding ovulation, which are the most fertile days of the cycle for trying to time intercourse.

For timing intercourse, it is advantageous to keep track of your cervical mucus changes so you can be warned of approaching ovulation. Note on your chart whether your mucus was dry (d), wet (w) or Spinn (s). As you watch your charts over several months, you can see how the mucus changes correlate with the temperature change. Maybe you always seem to have 4-5 days of dry, then 4-5 days of wetness building up, then 2 days of Spinn and then drying up. This knowledge of your usual mucus pattern will tell you when ovulation and the temp shift is imminent, and intercourse should happen if possible.

Watch your mucus for Spinn as it will indicate your day(s) of maximum fertility. It would be a good idea for you and your husband to avoid making love for about five days before you expect the shift from infertile to fertile mucus, in order for him to have a good, high sperm count. This will be during the time your mucus is building up in quantity and becoming liquid. When the mucus gets thin and clear, make love approximately every other day (for high sperm counts). If you have several days of Spinn, make love every other day throughout. If you do not get any Spinn (some women don't), then use the days of maximum clear mucus. Your temps will be low. Make love again as your temperature begins to ascend. The *last day* of Spinn is usually the day before ovulation, and is the *most fertile day of your cycle*. If you make love then, you will have fresh young sperm waiting for the egg to emerge. You can then make love freely until about five days before you next expect fertile mucus.

If your husband has had a sperm count and it is 50 million per cc or above, there is no need to abstain to save sperm; just look for the fertile mucus and other signs of ovulation, so you don't miss it. If the count is 30-50 million, it may help to save sperm, especially if there might be a female subfertility factor. If the count is under 30 million, abstention to concentrate the sperm count would definitely be of value.

There are a few other signs of ovulation or approaching ovulation. Many women notice that their breasts become tender and a little larger around ovulation as well as before their period. In fact, some women have this tenderness from the time of ovulation until their next period (if it is severe, vitamin E will often help).

Some women notice that they feel a little emotional or vulnerable around ovulation. You may also perceive a pain in your lower abdomen at this time. Doctors call it "mittelschmirtz"—German for "pain in the middle." It can be a sharp pain or dull and achey. It is probably a reaction to fluid flowing into the abdominal cavity.

Around the time you expect ovulation, see if you find yourself more sexually attracted to your mate than usual. Pay attention! This special sexy time is nature's way of encouraging the continuance of the species. It is a periodic "procreative urge" controlled by hormones. Follow your instincts.

If these timing guidelines would have you abstain from making love (to save sperm) at a time when you are feeling this particularly intense attraction, then by all means, ignore them. Don't get caught up in "rules" at the expense of what may be a deep instinctual message.

A few timing examples:

This woman knew from previous charts that she usually ovulated around the 13th-16th day. She also knew that her temperature rise (signaling that ovulation had passed) was usually preceded by 3 or 4 days of Spinn mucus. So they started refraining from making love around the 7th day in order to have some sperm saved up by the time her mucus turned to Spinn. When she noticed Spinn, they made love once every other day until the temperature rose and the mucus dried up. After her temp went up, they were free to make love until about the 7th day of the next cycle.

Basal Temperature Chart

Chart number_____

Name _____

Month(s) _____

Year_____

Shortest Previous Cycle_____

Longest Previous Cycle_____

Length of this cycle **28**

Day of month / week

Temperature

99.5
99.4
99.3
99.2
99.1
99.0
98.9
98.8
98.7
98.6
98.5
98.4
98.3
98.2
98.1
98.0
97.9
97.8
97.7
97.6
97.5
97.4
97.3
97.2
97.1
97.0

PERIOD

Mucus, other observations and disturbances

dry
dry
tacky
milky
wet, clear
spinn
spinn
spinn
dry
dry
tacky
dry

This woman has only had one day of Spinn mucus, sometimes only an increased wetness. They start making love every other day when her mucus gets clear and fluid, and continue until her temperature is high.

Basal Temperature Chart

Chart number_____

Name _____ Shortest Previous Cycle_____

Month(s) _____ Longest Previous Cycle_____

Year_____ Length of this cycle **31**

Day of month

week

Temperature

| 1 | 2 | 3 | 4 | 5 | 6 | 7 | 8 | 9 | 10 | 11 | 12 | 13 | 14 | 15 | 16 | 17 | 18 | 19 | 20 | 21 | 22 | 23 | 24 | 25 | 26 | 27 | 28 | 29 | 30 | 31 | 32 | 33 | 34 | 35 | 36 | 37 | 38 | 39 | 40 | 41 | 42 |

99.5
99.4
99.3
99.2
99.1
99.0
98.9
98.8
98.7
98.6
98.5
98.4
98.3
98.2
98.1
98.0
97.9
97.8
97.7
97.6
97.5
97.4
97.3
97.2
97.1
97.0

PERIOD

XXXX

Mucus, other observations and disturbances

dry
dry
dry
white, tacky
white, wet
clear, wet
wet
wet
spinn
wet
dry
dry

This woman has very short cycles most of the time. Her temperature is usually on the rise by the 10th or 11th day, indicating that ovulation has already passed. If she thought she was ovulating and fertile around the 14th day, she would be very mistaken. She usually ovulates around day 9 or 10 with 21-24 day cycles. Here she probably ovulated on day 8 or 9. To try to conceive she will make love almost every day from the 6th day of her period (and cycle) until her temp is high.

This woman became pregnant this cycle. She knew she was pregnant when her temperature remained elevated for longer than 20 days.

Basal Temperature Chart

Chart number_____

Name _____ Shortest Previous Cycle_____

Month(s) _____ · _____ Longest Previous Cycle_____

Year_____ Length of this cycle_____

Day of month / week

Temperature

99.5	
99.4	
99.3	
99.2	
99.1	
99.0	
98.9	
98.8	
98.7	
98.6	
98.5	
98.4	
98.3	
98.2	
98.1	
98.0	
97.9	
97.8	
97.7	
97.6	
97.5	
97.4	
97.3	
97.2	
97.1	
97.0	

Mucas, other observations and disturbances

spinn
spinn
wet
tacky
tacky
dry
dry

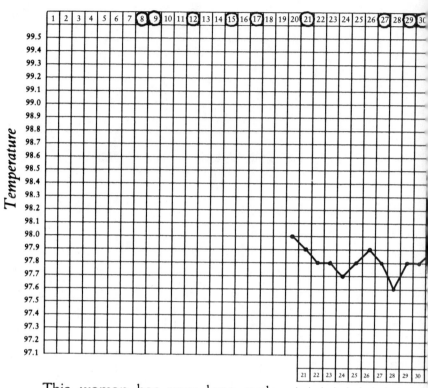

This woman has very long cycles, usually 50-70 days. She doesn't take her temperature until around day 20. Since she has such variation in cycle length, they can't really figure out which days, prior to the appearance of mucus, to abstain. So they can't try to save up sperm. But she *can* watch carefully for the appearance of wet and Spinn mucus, and try to arrange some loving for that time. Note they made love at the appearance of some wet mucus on days 27 and 35 (but the temp didn't rise those times).

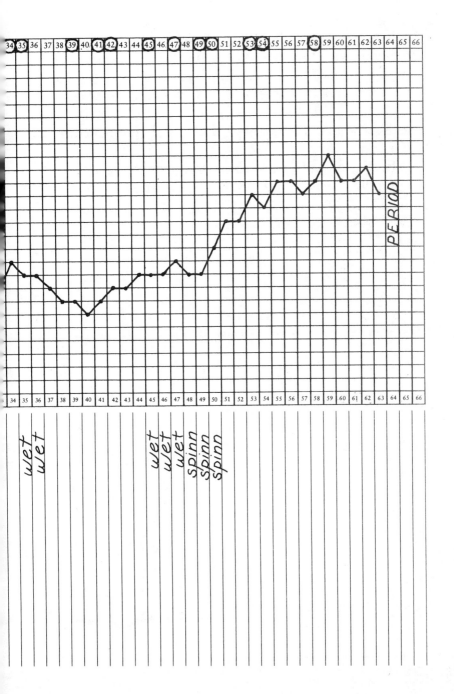

If scheduling intercourse is ruining your sex life, making you feel pressured, unspontaneous, desperate, turned off...DON'T DO IT! Believe me, it's not worth it if it causes tension or friction. You might do better to let nature take its course once you have established ovulation by the basal temperature method.

But if you both want to try to have intercourse at optimum times, and avoid it sometimes for an increased sperm count, then good luck on your cooperative journey.

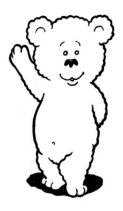

one last pitch for

FERTILITY AWARENESS

Whether you are coping with established subfertility factors, coming to peace with medically confirmed infertility, or just wondering why the expected conception hasn't happened yet, you will gain many personal benefits from monitoring the signs of your own reproductive cycle. Even if you only watch your mucus changes and/or chart your temperature for a few months, you will be surprised at how familiar and "in charge" you will feel with your body. It's a liberating feeling to be able to observe ovulation approach and pass, and to accurately predict one's periods.

Through fertility awareness, you can observe your cyclic changes from a more objective viewpoint. If you tend to get a little insecure or touchy around ovulation or the day or two before your period, you can notice it's "that time" and remind yourself that you are experiencing hormonal fluctuations, and things will feel better shortly. Most women experience mood changes because of hormones, but these are especially difficult times for women anxious to become pregnant or coming to terms with infertility.

It is easier to be graceful under the pressure if you are in touch with the orderly and somewhat predictable events of your female cycle.

CONCLUSION

Does it sound a little overwhelming: the fertility questions, the hormone interactions, the tests, the uncertainty?

Many of the conditions and suggestions described in this book will not apply to each of you because there is such a wide spectrum of causes of subfertility and infertility. You as an individual and a couple, have your own special set of circumstances. If you have blocked tubes, your options and prognosis are different from someone with few periods, or endometriosis, or a seriously impaired sperm count.

Some of you will conceive through increased fertility awareness, whether you have a "normal" reproductive potential and merely poor timing of intercourse, or a *reduced* but not absent fertility— such as a moderately low sperm count, rare ovulation, poor cervical mucus, or a combination of these lesser factors. These conditions can sometimes be overcome by paying attention to the fertile time, and strategic saving up of sperm.

Some of you may conceive through medical intervention such as drugs, hormones, or surgery. You too may increase your chances through fertility awareness.

And some of you, dear friends, will probably not conceive at all, for reasons such as azoospermia (no sperm at all), severe endometriosis, irreparable scarred tubes, or too strong a combination of subfertile factors such as oligospermia (very few sperm) paired with inhospitable mucus, etc. Often, if you can know and understand the reason why you cannot conceive, or at least determine that after much investigation the mystery is not to be solved, it can be easier to live with the situation and accept a different assignment in life.

If children are essential to you, perhaps you can love and cherish someone else's child, who through unfortunate circumstances is alone. It is true that the adoption lines are long, and babies are scarce, but every state has its forgotten children, its "difficult to place" children who need to be claimed, loved and raised.

INDEX

About the Author:

Margaret Nofziger was born in San Francisco, California in 1946. She is married and the mother of two children. Her first child was born after 8 years of apparent infertility, and the second after three years of trying.

Ms. Nofziger authored a best-selling book on family planning which has been translated into six languages.

Basal Temperature Chart

Chart number_____

Name _____ Shortest Previous Cycle_____

Month(s) _____ Longest Previous Cycle_____

Year_____ Length of this cycle_____

Day of month / week

	1	2	3	4	5	6	7	8	9	10	11	12	13	14	15	16	17	18	19	20	21	22	23	24	25	26	27	28	29	30	31	32	33	34	35	36	37	38	39	40	41	42

Temperature

99.5
99.4
99.3
99.2
99.1
99.0
98.9
98.8
98.7
98.6
98.5
98.4
98.3
98.2
98.1
98.0
97.9
97.8
97.7
97.6
97.5
97.4
97.3
97.2
97.1
97.0

Mucus, other observations and disturbances